HERBAL MEDICINE FOR THE MENOPAUSE

by Andrew Chevallier BA FNIMH

Published by
Amberwood Publishing Ltd
Guildford, England

CONTENTS

About The Author

Andrew Chevallier is an experienced medical herbalist and fellow of The National Institute of Medical Herbalists with practices in Norwich and London. He is a Senior Lecturer in Herbal Medicine (p/t) at Middlesex University and has recently been involved in researching the use of herbal medicines for menopausal symptoms. He has written several books on herbs and herbalism, including Herbal First Aid , Herbal Teas and 50 Vital Herbs published by Amberwood Publishing and The Encyclopedia of Medicinal Plants, which has sold over a million copies worldwide.

Note to Reader

Foreword

The menopause is a major transition in the life of a woman, taking her from her childbearing years into what should be a time of great satisfaction. At this stage in her life, it is likely that she will have the benefit of years of accumulated wisdom, increased financial stability, now that she no longer has to meet the demands of her children, and more leisure time to enjoy. My experience of helping thousands of women through their menopause over the last eighteen years, confirms that this phase is only likely to be enjoyable when good health prevails.

For approximately three-quarters of women consuming a Western diet, the menopause brings a collection of unwanted and persistent symptoms including hot flushes, night sweats, resulting in insomnia, dry vagina and aches and pains, leaving them feeling a shadow of their former selves.

Most doctors are willing to prescribe Hormone Replacement Therapy in order to control the symptoms of the menopause, as this is the approach with which they are most familiar. However, research shows that up to two-thirds of women who try HRT, come off it within the first year, due to side effects or dissatisfaction, and they are often then left to fend for themselves.

What is not widely appreciated, is that there is a scientifically based alternative, which does not involve taking hormone therapy. Instead making specific dietary changes and taking supplements, including a wide range of herbs, can alleviate symptoms of the menopause.

Science now confirms that herbal medicine has a great deal to offer women at the time of their menopause, without having the side effects associated with HRT. Specific herbs have been clearly shown to influence hormone balance, whilst others have little effect at this time. Andrew Chevallier, a Fellow and Past President of the National Institute of Medical Herbalists, is well qualified to interpret the science into a workable and useable plan. He provides an easy to understand reference guide to tried and tested herbs according to symptoms. Plus clear guidelines are provided on self-help measures and he draws a line in the sand indicating when it becomes advisable to consult a qualified practitioner. *Herbal Medicine for the Menopause* is a valuable asset to add to your bookshelf.

Maryon Stewart
Founder – *Women's Nutritional Advisory Service*
November 2001

1 | Introduction

About this book

This book sets out to try and provide the essential information you need on herbs and the menopause, for you to make sensible decisions about whether herbal treatment is right for you; and assuming that it is, what herbs or extracts to take, how much and when. The advice given is based both on longstanding traditional use and scientific research, where available. A section at the end of the book gives suggestions for further reading and other helpful sources.

As a practical book *Herbal Medicine for the Menopause* contains useful information on: -

- How to select over the counter herbs and herbal extracts

- How to use herbal remedies to support good health and hormonal balance before and during the menopause

- How to use herbal remedies to relieve menopausal symptoms

- General advice, including diet, on promoting health during the menopause

- Advice on herbal alternatives to HRT, and what you can do to help maintain healthy bones and joints into later life

- When to consider seeing a medical herbalist for professional advice if conventional or self-treatment has not helped.

This practical advice reflects the contemporary use of plant medicines around the world to treat and relieve menopausal problems. Many of these herbal medicines have a traditional use going back for hundreds and in some cases thousands of years. Some examples – all looked at in detail later in the book – give a glimpse of the many herbs used traditionally by women across the world to improve their health and quality of life during the menopause.

In Russia and the middle east, liquorice root has been used traditionally as a good tonic treatment for symptoms such as hot flushing and tiredness linked to the menopause. It has a powerful anti-inflammatory action, is mildly oestrogenic and strengthens adrenal gland function.

In China and the far east, *dong quai* (Chinese Angelica) has been taken for at least 5,000 years and continues to be taken on a daily basis by hundreds of millions of women. Traditionally being thought to enhance vitality and libido, it has constituents that support the circulation and liver function.

In Europe, sage tea is an ancient remedy for hot flushing and night sweats, now being researched in detail and found to have oestrogenic, antioxidant and tonic activity.

These examples give a taste of the benefits that herbal medicines can offer, and the scale with which they have been used over the centuries for their hormonal and tonic effects.

When taking herbal medicines it is important to remember that they *are* medicines and can produce side effects, although the evidence – from long-term traditional use and modern scientific investigation – shows that provided they are used with sufficient care side effects are rare and almost always mild in character.

Many issues affect the safety and effectiveness of herbal medicines – dosage, the type of preparation or extract, the length of treatment, the combination of herbs employed and possible interactions with conventional medicines. As a result, it is often better to consult a qualified medical herbalist for advice and a prescription (see page 68), though in many situations – and this includes mild to moderate menopausal symptoms – self-treatment makes good sense and is likely to be effective.

Troublesome problems such as hot flushing, low mood and poor sleep can frequently be relieved with herbal self-treatment. When combined with a good diet, appropriate exercise and a positive outlook on life, such self-care can help to improve vitality and quality of life and usher in new opportunities.

2 | Herbs and hormonal balance

"Of one thing we are certain, and that is, that the change will take place without danger if the body is in health."

Skelton's Family Medical Adviser 1873

Hormonal balance

Throughout life, hormone levels and hormonal balance changes. Sometimes the changes are slight, sometimes major, but usually such changes follow the body's unconscious wisdom – a pattern that is as deep as life itself and which carries us literally from the womb to the grave.

In our teens we grow into biological adults, our bodies responding so rapidly to changing levels of sex hormones that adolescents are as likely to feel disturbed and out of control, as they are excited at 'growing up'. For women, from adolescence to menopause, hormonal change is the norm: a regular menstrual cycle bringing rhythmical change throughout the body. During the 30's and onwards levels of sex hormones decline (in men and women), leading in the late 40's to what may be the first signs of menopause – irregular menstrual cycles with unpredictable, heavy bleeding – as oestrogen and progesterone release by the ovaries reduces.

At this time, the body's inner wisdom instinctively moves towards a new hormonal balance, compensating for reduced ovarian hormones by increasing the production of weaker oestrogens from the adrenal glands and in fatty tissue. Eventually, by the early to mid 50's the menstrual cycle ends and a new hormonal balance is established. From this time onwards oestrogen levels within the body gradually increase.

The major hormonal changes that occur at the menopause do not however always go smoothly and the body can find it hard to arrive at a new state of balance. Hormone levels, principally oestrogen, can fluctuate up and down causing some of the common menopausal symptoms. In fact, poor hormonal balance is often more of a problem than the lowered level of hormones that occurs naturally.

Where levels of ovarian hormones fluctuate widely, hormonal balance throughout the body – maintained by the central nervous and endocrine system, including the thyroid and adrenal glands – can be put under pressure. Not surprisingly, such imbalance can produce symptoms reflecting this hormonal 'dis-stress': from hot flushing and disturbed sleep to worry, depression, disorientation and poor concentration. Re-establishing hormonal balance – restoring equilibrium within the body and mind, and strengthening adrenal and other glandular function – is the key to relieving these symptoms.

Oestrogen influences all types of tissue within the body and the decline in oestrogen levels at the menopause is linked to changes throughout the body, particularly in the breasts, vagina, bones, blood vessels, skin, and the digestive and urinary tracts. These changes are natural and normal, though they can lead to problems such as vaginal dryness, urinary incontinence and osteoporosis. However, when one looks closely at the reasons why women develop such health problems, there are often other pre-existing health factors present such as long-term stress, poor nutritional state or low body weight.

Improving your diet, doing a bit more exercise and adjusting some aspects of your lifestyle can often help to prevent the onset of symptoms which are traditionally associated with the menopause. In some societies, notably Japan, the traditional diet – rich in minerals, plant oestrogens and polyunsaturated fats – not only helps women to have a symptom-free menopause but to live longer, and everyone today recognises that making changes to one's diet and lifestyle can lead to a marked improvement in health. Alongside these self-help approaches, there are a number of safe and effective herbal medicines that can bring real relief to menopausal problems.

Herbs for hormonal balance

Several herbal remedies – Linseed, Agnus Castus and Black Cohosh are key examples – have direct but subtle hormonal activity within the body, and are able to support a return to hormonal balance at the menopause.

Most hormonally-active herbs are oestrogenic (see Chapter 3 on phytoestrogens) and encourage hormonal balance at the menopause by increasing oestrogen levels. Linseed – taken as food or medicine – falls within this category, as it contains unusually high levels of lignans, oestrogenic compounds that exert a mild hormonal activity within the body. Taken long term, Linseed and other oestrogenic foods/herbs, such as Soya, help the body to adjust to lowered oestrogen levels. Other herbs with established oestrogenic activity include: Fenugreek, Hops and Sage.

A small category of herbs have a progesterone rather than an oestrogen-type activity. Agnus Castus is not directly progesterogenic but acts on the pituitary gland at the base of the brain, indirectly increasing release of progesterone by the ovaries and promoting hormonal balance during the menstrual cycle. Agnus Castus can therefore help to improve menstrual irregularity, and relieve the breast tenderness, fluid retention and heavy bleeding that can occur a year or so before menopause. It is also prescribed by medical herbalists to promote hormonal balance during the menopause, complementing other herbs such as Black Cohosh. Used in this way it can form part of a long term approach to treating menopausal problems.

A third category of herbs influence hormonal balance indirectly and one could almost say that strictly speaking they do not have hormonal activity! Until recently, Black Cohosh was thought to have oestrogenic activity, but research now suggests that it works by influencing neurotransmitters within the central nervous system – probably in the area of the brain close to the pituitary gland. Several clinical trials have shown that Black Cohosh is an effective treatment for menopausal symptoms including hot flushing, sweating, headache, dizziness and tinnitus (ringing in the ears). In one 1982 trial, 80% of women experienced notable improvement in symptoms, in about 45% of cases the symptoms cleared altogether. In a 1998 trial, improvement in symptoms occurred within two weeks and after 6 months approximately 90% of the women taking Black Cohosh extract had experienced a reduction in symptoms. Though there is little knowledge of how the herb works within the body, there is growing evidence to show that it is an effective remedy for common menopausal symptoms.

Menopausal symptoms

The following symptoms – hot flushing and vaginal dryness – are thought to be the only ones *directly* linked to lowered oestrogen levels. Other symptoms that occur at the menopause may have a hormonal element but are probably due to other factors as well – such as poor circulation, nervous exhaustion, stress levels, infection and so on. The herbs listed are the one's most likely to be of help – look them up in the main section for more details.

Hot flushing and night sweats

- Symptoms of heat and flushing across the head and upper body, which can last from a few seconds to 30 minutes, are experienced by 80% of menopausal women and occur anything from once a week to many times a day. Sweating, especially at night, often accompanies hot flushing, which is thought to be caused by bursts of luteinising hormone released by the pituitary gland as it tries to stimulate ovarian hormone production. In most cases hot flushes last for less than two years with only a few women experiencing them for more than five years.

- *Worsened by*: alcohol, coffee, tea, other hot drinks and food, hot spices, stress, shock and anxiety.

- *Relieved by*: cool drinks, wearing layers of clothes that can be adapted to temperature changes (also at night), foods with oestrogenic activity.

- *Key herbs*: Black Cohosh, Red Clover, Sage, Liquorice.

Vaginal dryness

- From menopause, the walls of the vagina gradually become thinner, drier and less elastic and more prone to infection. These changes can make sexual intercourse uncomfortable or painful and many women find it helpful to lubricate the vagina (use water-soluble lubricants as they help reduce the chance of infection). Some local applications can help to improve the tone of vaginal tissue.

- *Worsened by*: lack of oestrogen-rich foods in diet, possibly by lack of exercise and non-active sexual life.

- *Relieved by*: locally applied water-based ointments and creams – Marigold/Calendula cream is antiseptic, healing and mildly oestrogenic and makes a good lubricant; oestrogenic foods and herbs.

- *Key herbs*: Fenugreek, Chinese Angelica, Wild Yam, Agnus Castus.

Many different factors, including lowered hormonal levels, may lie behind the following symptoms. Treatment needs to look at the whole range of possible causes:

Anxiety, nervousness and irritability

- Anxiety, as everyone knows, can occur at any time, though hormonal factors may play a part when it occurs at the menopause. A wave of anxiety often accompanies a hot flush, and may feel quite different from anxiety produced by worry or stress. Anxiety and irritability are also more likely to occur when the body is out of balance – whether the imbalance is fluctuating blood sugar levels or oestrogen levels or some other hormonal disorder. In each case, a sense of one's body being beyond control produces a stressful situation, typically undermining self-confidence and causing worry, nervousness and irritability. Working to support better balance within the body is an important part of relieving these problems: start doing some/all of the things listed below and seek out those people who give you sound emotional support and advice.
- *Worsened by*: coffee and tea, alcohol, chocolate and sugar-rich foods, irregular eating and poor diet, lack of exercise, lack of relaxation, stress and emotional states involving fear and insecurity, poor or inadequate sleep.
- *Relieved by*: regular healthy eating that supports balanced blood sugar levels, good quality sleep, regular relaxation and exercise including deep breathing exercises and yoga, emotional balance and mediation, B vitamins, foods such as oats.
- *Key herbs*: Kava Kava, Scullcap, Motherwort.

Breast tenderness

- A common pre-menstrual symptom, especially when close to the menopause, breast tenderness and swelling suggests that there is congestion in the body, particularly within the lymphatic system that drains fluid lying outside the arteries and veins. Lymph nodes can become blocked so that there is poor flow through them – dietary changes and more exercise are a good starting point in treating this problem, but if it persists see a medical herbalist or your GP.

- *Worsened by*: coffee and tea, alcohol, salt, poor diet, lack of exercise, nervous tension and anxiety.
- *Relieved by*: regular healthy eating, plenty of water, regular relaxation and exercise, foods such as carrot, celery, cabbage – also as juices.
- *Key herbs*: Agnus Castus, Lady's Mantle, Marigold/Calendula.

Depression

- Depression is a catch-all word that covers everything from 'feeling out of sorts' to severe depression, where life no longer feels worth living. If you are suffering from severe, or moderate, depression you need professional help and should contact your GP, a medical herbalist or other suitable healthcare professional. For less severe depression around the menopause try and see if there are factors in your life causing depression – the more you can do to ease burdensome problems the better. Where this is not possible, be kind to yourself, talk to friends, nourish yourself – with food and 'soul' food. Where there is a hormonal aspect to the depression, consider herbs such as Black Cohosh, Sage and Red Clover. Depression is also commonly linked to long term anxiety and nervous exhaustion. A plan that helps to restore vitality and reconnect you with the 'spice of life' might include: eating better, doing some regular exercise and deep breathing exercises, finding time to get out – perhaps to a social event or a yoga class, and taking herbs such as St. John's Wort.
- *Worsened by*: negative thoughts, poor self-care, poor sleep, lack of exercise, alcohol, poor diet and lack of omega-3 oils and B vitamins.
- *Relieved by*: more or less the reverse of the previous section! Positive thoughts, good quality sleep, regular exercise, good diet including plenty of whole grains and fish.
- *Key herbs*: St. John's Wort, Kava Kava, Liquorice.

Dry skin

- The skin gets slowly drier with age and nourishing it with oils is a pleasant and relaxing activity. The skin needs plenty of water to keep hydrated so drink at least 1 litre of water a day. Bathing is good but don't use lots of soap. After a bath or shower apply wheatgerm or vitamin E oil or creams to dry areas of skin. Other skin-nourishing oils include: avocado (you can mash it and apply fresh!) jojoba and sweet almond. Olive oil makes a good soak for a dry scalp – leave on for 30-40 minutes before washing out.

- *Worsened by*: smoking, alcohol, lack of oestrogen-rich foods in diet, lack of essential fatty acids.
- *Relieved by*: locally applied oils and creams, supplementing with omega-3 and -6 oils.
- *Key herbs*: Liquorice (orally), Wheatgerm and other oils on the skin.

Headaches

- Headaches can be troublesome during the menopause and accompany hot flushing and poor sleep. As hormonal factors may be a contributory factor it is worth trying herbs such as Black Cohosh and Sage, which can bring significant relief. If this does not help, try to reduce stress levels, relax and improve diet - all the familiar suggestions! Cutting out foods commonly linked with headaches and migraines – alcohol, caffeine, chocolate, oranges, cheese, etc. – can be helpful.
- *Worsened by*: Physical and emotional tension, postural problems, poor diet, lack of exercise.
- *Relieved by*: relaxation and relaxing exercise, drinking more water, eating regular meals, good quality sleep.
- *Key herbs*: Scullcap, Kava Kava.

Heavy menstrual bleeding and flooding

- During the 1-3 years before the menopause the menstrual cycle generally becomes irregular and periods can become unusually heavy. Over a third of women in their late 40's have shorter cycles which skip ovulation, leading to heavier bleeding. Heavy bleeding can also happen when the cycle is longer than usual and the period is delayed. If bleeding occurs between periods or continues on without stopping see your GP or medical herbalist.
- *Worsened by*: alcohol, lack of exercise, poor circulation, anaemia.
- *Relieved by*: Nettle tea.
- *Key herbs*: Lady's Mantle, Agnus Castus.

Poor sleep

- For sleep disturbed by hot flushing and night sweats, see section above, as well as this one. Where poor sleep results from anxiety or depression, daytime problems need attention as well. Doctors talk about 'sleep hygiene' and this is a useful idea – taking care not to eat or to drink alcohol late, allowing time to unwind and relax in the evening (not watching the horror movie on the television!), perhaps doing some yoga or meditation, keeping your bedroom free from clutter and making it as restful a place as possible. Establishing a regular pattern in going to bed also helps to re-establish regular sleeping.

- *Worsened by*: eating late, caffeine in evening, more than about 2 units of alcohol, being 'keyed up' and mentally overactive, lack of regularity in evening and going to bed.

- *Relieved by*: better relaxation, physical exercise during the day, relaxing exercise in the evening, meditation.

- *Key herbs*: Kava Kava, Scullcap, Hops.

Urinary incontinence

- Tissue in the urinary tract changes with age and sometimes leaves women susceptible to incontinence, particularly if certain chronic illnesses or urinary infections are also present. Coughing, laughing, lifting heavy objects and exercises that put pressure on the bladder may cause small amounts of urine to leak. Incontinence is usually treatable and is not a normal part of ageing. Doing regular pelvic floor exercises is one of the most useful treatments as it strengthens the ligaments that keep the bladder and womb in place. Kava Kava can be very helpful for bladder irritability.

- *Worsened by*: lack of regular exercise, poor diet – especially sugar, and acidic foods, anxiety and tension.

- *Relieved by*: regular non-stressful exercise: walking, swimming, yoga, etc., changing diet – increase lemon and carrots, barley and oats, relaxation.

- *Key herbs*: Cranberry, Kava Kava.

3 | Phytoestrogens and HRT

Herbal remedies are able to help at the menopause in several ways and their ability to influence hormone levels – in particular oestrogen levels – is by now fairly well understood. Knowing a little about how herbs work hormonally and interact with the body's own hormones increases the chances of using them successfully.

Phytoestrogens or plant-oestrogens

Phytoestrogens are naturally-occurring plant substances that act like oestrogen within the body. Their strength of activity has been estimated at around 1/100th that of the body's oestrogen. Many plants used as foods and medicines contain such compounds. Red Clover and Soya contain isoflavones; Linseed contains lignans. All are thought to complement the body's oestrogen levels – increasing oestrogenic activity when oestrogen levels are low e.g. at the menopause, while some also appear to reduce oestrogen activity when levels are too high, as can occur e.g. with fibroids. As a result phytoestrogen-rich plants may well be useful in a wide range of hormonally-related health problems, although they have most value in supporting and maintaining hormonal balance around the menopause.

Phytoestrogens are oestrogenic but they have a number of other beneficial effects within the body as well. They are antioxidant and protect tissue from free-radical damage, help to counter bone loss and heart disease, and in some cases have anti-inflammatory activity as well. Their range of activity within the body is not yet fully understood.

Many plants also contain compounds which indirectly influence oestrogen levels within the body. Sterols are common plant constituents found for example in Oats and Nettle root; the less common but more medicinally potent steroidal and triterpenoid saponins are found in herbs such as Ginseng, Liquorice and Wild Yam. It seems that the body is able to use such compounds in a variety of ways, depending on the hormonal circumstances present at the time. From the menopause onwards, such herbs can be used to support oestrogen levels within the body.

Soya is the best known food with significant levels of phytoestrogens but all beans and lentils, many root vegetables and a multitude of other foods such as seeds and wholegrains, also contain worthwhile levels (see section on diet in next chapter). Herbs with notable phytoestrogenic activity include Fennel, Hops, Liquorice, Red Clover and Sage.

For a long time it has been recognised that in several Asian countries and especially in Japan, where the diet traditionally includes lots of phytoestrogen-rich foods, particularly soya and mung beans, women are less prone to menopausal problems such as hot flushing. Women in these societies are also likely to live longer and to have lower rates of heart disease, osteoporosis and breast cancer than women in the west.

As this protective role of phytoestrogens has become better known, supplementing with phytoestrogenic foods and herbs has become more and more popular in the west. The benefits of an increased intake of foods like soya and lentils – as part of a healthy 'whole' food diet – are clear. When it comes to supplements which deliver highly concentrated levels of phytoestrogens, e.g. Red Clover or Soya extracts, the situation is perhaps less straightforward.

Phytoestrogens do not occur on their own in nature, rarely being found at concentrations above 2.5% in plants. This means that 97.5% of the remainder of the plant is non-oestrogenic, and that phytoestrogens naturally occur well-diluted! Eating phytoestrogen-rich foods or taking oestrogenic herbs at normal concentrations provides phytoestrogens in their natural context and in the form that they have been traditionally used in the past. As a result one can be fairly sure that such foods and herbs are almost entirely safe.

Concentrated extracts can contain much higher levels of naturally-occurring phytoestrogens – sometimes being concentrated 50 times or more – and may prove more effective in relieving menopausal symptoms in the short term, though as logic would suggest, being more concentrated they may also be more likely to cause side effects. As the concentration of phytoestrogens increases so the complex mix of other 'background' constituents is reduced and the product becomes increasingly unlike its natural counterpart – the dried herb and simple extracts. Such concentrated extracts can provide valuable *short-term* treatment (maximum 3 months) and are recommended if normal concentrations of oestrogenic foods and herbs fail to ease menopausal symptoms. Nevertheless, foods, supplements and herbal products in a form close to their natural state are the preferred form of treatment.

Foods vs. supplements

Until recently soya and phytoestrogens were universally seen as good nutrition and good preventative medicine. Rest assured, soya *does* make good food – but at high doses and when not fermented, it reduces the ability of the digestive system to absorb several minerals, including iron, and vitamins A, B, C and E. In Japan, the traditional diet has always included plenty of seaweed – rich in iron and many trace minerals – as a staple alongside soya, which people have thought makes up for the reduced absorption linked with the high soy intake.

In the case of phytoestrogens, the recommended dosage is around 40mg a day – equivalent to about 20g a day of soya protein (tofu). It may well be fine to take much higher doses than this for several months or longer as food (the Japanese on average eat about 75g of soy protein a day), but it is questionable whether highly concentrated phytoestrogenic extracts of Soya or Red Clover are advisable for long term use.

What about progesterone?

So far as is known, no plants contain progesterone, the hormone that supports conception and works with oestrogen in regulating the menstrual cycle. Claims for 'natural progesterone' derived from plants are misleading. If one looks into it, 'natural' progesterone is produced in a laboratory from chemicals extracted from plants – dioscine from Wild Yam – and is in most respects identical to progesterone that has been artificially produced.

A few medicinal plants have a progesterogenic activity, but none contain progesterone. Agnus Castus is the best known, but Vervain (*Verbena officinalis*) also has some progesterogenic activity.

Natural alternatives or HRT?

As one might expect, there is no simple answer to this question, and trying to find one's way through the complex arguments for and against

HRT and natural alternatives is far from easy. There are a number of points that can be made that may make it more straightforward to decide what is best for you:

- Even those who support the use of HRT rarely go so far as to say that all women should take it. There are doctors who argue for this but they are in a minority. Medical herbalists argue that HRT is worth considering only if you have tried dietary and herbal approaches and these have been unsuccessful. In any case, the return of periods, possible weight gain and an increased risk of breast cancer are commonly recognised as disincentives, when considering whether to take HRT. There may be situations where taking HRT is advisable, e.g. where there are early signs of osteoporosis or a family history of it, but even in situations like this the evidence is not clear-cut.

- There has been much publicity about the safety of HRT: there are increased risks of developing breast, ovarian and endometrial cancer, gallstones, thrombosis and lupus. Other associated problems include raised blood pressure, headaches, migraines, dizziness and fibrocystic breast disease. These risks are counter-balanced by a reduction in the chances of developing osteoporosis, Alzheimer's disease and heart and circulatory disease. It is not clear whether the reduction in risk (especially of osteoporosis) continues after stopping HRT or occurs only while taking it. Herbal alternatives to HRT are highly unlikely to cause serious side effects and it is *probably* the case that herbs can be as effective as HRT as a preventative, but this is *not* clinically proven. Evidence suggests that Black Cohosh, and phytoestrogen-containing plants such as Soya, Linseed and Red Clover can act like HRT in protecting against osteoporosis and cardio-vascular disease, though the research that will confirm or deny this is yet to be done. Ginkgo has been clinically shown to prevent the onset of Alzheimer's disease.

- As with other aspects of health, treatment should match your needs. Whenever possible, try dietary and herbal approaches first, as these work with the body and can improve health overall. Even with fairly severe menopausal symptoms natural treatments can bring relief quite quickly. Giving yourself 8-10 weeks on the recommendations made in this book is generally enough time to see whether treatment is effective in relieving menopausal symptoms, though in more severe cases it is advisable to see a qualified medical herbalist, who can provide advice and treatment to fit your individual needs. When taking herbs and supplements for *long term* prevention of osteoporosis, etc., rather than for immediate relief – take lower doses, perhaps even 50% of the normal recommended dosage.

- Not everyone will automatically benefit from herbs, any more than they do from HRT. It is also possible for side effects to occur, though these are almost always minor and disappear on stopping treatment.

- Although the word 'philosophy' is *rarely* used in conventional medicine, people do seek medical treatment that accords with their view of life. Herbal medicine's philosophy is that in working with nature, in harmony with body, mind and spirit – you have a better chance of restoring health and vitality. For herbalists, HRT (and to a lesser extent, extracts where the herb is concentrated 50-fold or more) is best avoided because it overrides the body/mind/spirit's capacity to self-repair and to heal. However much we all want it, health (as opposed to relief of symptoms) does not usually come out of a bottle or tablet jar. Attention to diet, exercise and one's emotional life is often more important!

4 | Staying healthy in mid-life

The basic 'ground rules' for health do not change through life – everyone needs good clean air and water, adequate nutrition and exercise, care and love – though the precise details of what helps to maintain good health do change according to age. A simple, common sense approach to diet and exercise, along with a positive outlook and a willingness to be kind to oneself and to others will provide most of what is required for good health in mid-life, particularly around the menopause.

Dietary Advice

- *Try and eat food that is as close to its natural state as possible – either as natural as you can find it, or as natural as you can bear to eat it!*
  By and large the more processed a food is the more it will have lost its nutritional goodness. Eating wholemeal bread will provide a significantly greater input of vitamins, minerals, oils and fibre than bread made from refined or bleached flour. At the same time, foods close to their natural state are less likely to have been tampered with and do not contain large quantities of unwanted additives, some with unwanted hormonal effects.

- *Take pleasure in what you eat and allow yourself to enjoy it.*
  As a counterbalance to the first recommendation, food is there to be savoured and enjoyed! Even foods which are not strictly good for you on a nutritional level may do you 'good' if eaten in small quantities. Being unnecessarily strict in one's diet – making a martyr of oneself – is counterproductive, unless there are specific reasons for excluding certain foods. Try to eat in a relaxed, unhurried way - which allows space and time for digestion to take place, and improves the absorption of nutrients in food.

- *Eat organically grown food where possible, especially apples, grapes, peppers, strawberries, root vegetables, dairy produce and meat.*

Although at present organic foods are more expensive than non-organic ones, there are compelling reasons for thinking that they are better value in the long term. Eating organic food reduces one's exposure to artificial pesticides and fertilisers and is likely to provide better nutrition. Broccoli grown in the UK in the 1940's typically contained at least twice as much iron as the broccoli that finds its way onto supermarket shelves today. Vegetables bred exclusively to look good on the shelves with no attention paid to nutritional value are one possible reason for this. The poor soil quality that goes with non-organic farming is almost certainly another. Organic foods require that life (microbes) is put back into the soil, for without them plants grown in the absence of artificial fertilisers are unable to draw minerals into their roots from the soil. The foods listed above – apples, etc. – are best eaten organically because when grown non-organically they are most likely to contain high levels of pesticides and fertilisers.

- *Eat more fruit, grains and vegetables, including beans, lentils and seeds.*
  Eating 5 pieces or portions of fruit and veg a day *is* a good idea. More is going to do you good – up to 75% of one's total intake. As the bulk of one's diet, these foods provide carbohydrates for energy, essential vitamins and minerals, and phytoestrogens. Many of them support a healthy heart and circulation and aid elimination. All members of the carrot family, e.g. parsnip, celery and fennel, all beans, lentils, seeds and grains contain phyoestrogens. Lastly, if you know a food does not agree with you – follow your instincts and avoid it rather than following advice from books such as this one!

- *Fats and oils – the good and the bad.*
  Without fats and oils we would not live long. At least 20% of our diet needs to be made up of fats and oils and contrary to popular opinion eating fats and oils does not automatically mean putting on weight. In fact, there is growing evidence that eating the right fats and oils in the right quantities promotes weight loss in the overweight. The key is quality. Many vegetable oils are extracted and processed in what can only be described as a disastrous way and, along with animal fats, should be avoided. Some seed and bean oils e.g. soya and sunflower, are naturally high in unstable polyunsaturated fatty acids. Treat them

carefully and these oils will provide vital nutrition for cell walls, especially in nerve tissue, for the skin and in many glands and hormonal processes, including the ovaries and adrenal glands. They will also help the body to cope more effectively with saturated fats. Treat them indifferently, paying little attention to retaining the special chemical bonds in these oils, and you destroy much of their nutritional value.

Fortunately, it is becoming easier to buy good quality oils. For stir-frying and wherever you need to apply direct heat, use organic virgin olive oil. For baking and on salads, use organic virgin soya or sunflower oils. It is also possible now to buy organic *non-hydrogenated* soya or sunflower margarines (avoid hydrogenated margarines of all kinds). These oils provide high levels of omega-6 oils.

Linseed/flaxseed oil is uniquely high in omega-3 oils and makes a valuable supplement alongside other good quality oils. Alternatively, eat oily fish – sardines, salmon, trout and mackerel – at least twice a week. These oils provide high levels of the rarer omega-3 oils. Many people are deficient in these oils and supplementation may be beneficial, especially during a difficult menopause.

- *Foods and drinks to avoid.*
Now for the bad news! Alcohol and caffeine-containing foods and drinks are 'anti-nutrients' providing little in the way of nutrition on the positive side of the balance sheet but using up precious resources as the body struggles to break them down and clear them from the system. Additionally, during the menopause they can act as triggers that set off hot flushes, though this can apply to hot drinks and spicy food in general. Somewhat jokingly they have been referred to as 'thermogenic insults' due to their destabilising effect on the body's temperature control system.

Alcohol is a depressant and in the medium term lowers mood – though that does not stop its very pleasant effects in the short term. Best advice if you are experiencing menopausal symptoms is to allow yourself the occasional glass or two but to try and restrict intake to 2 or 3 days a week at the most.

Coffee and tea in moderate amounts, say 1–3 cups a day in total, is fine if you are in good health, and there is evidence that this helps to keep one alert and in good spirits. In chronic health problems, caffeine is distinctly unhelpful, as its stimulant effect weakens an already under-resourced system.

Other foods which should be avoided altogether or kept to a low level include: sugar and sugar-rich foods; artificial sweeteners; deep fried foods including crisps, chips, etc; poor quality meat, such as burgers and pate; and junk food in general. Dairy produce is best kept at a moderate level.

Key essential nutrients

Vitamin B complex
B vitamins are essential nutrients for tissues throughout the body, though high levels are particularly required by nerve tissue. Different B vitamins are found naturally in many vegetables and grains. A good, balanced diet will normally ensure adequate intake. Take supplement as recommended – best when combined with Vitamin C.

Vitamin C
A key nutrient to maintain resistance to infection. A powerful antioxidant, vitamin C prevents cell breakdown and slows ageing. Lemon, grapefruit, peppers, parsley and all fresh fruit and vegetables are rich sources. As a supplement take up to 1g a day.

Vitamin E
Along with vitamin C, vitamin E is the most important antioxidant within the body, helping to protect tissue from free radical damage. The circulation, nerve and reproductive tissue are some of the most vulnerable to free radical damage. Increasing intake of vitamin E may help relieve hot flushes. Vitamin E is also a 'food' for the skin. Found in all seeds and whole grains: especially wheatgerm, sunflower seeds, oats. As a supplement recommended dosage is 400-1000 i.u. a day.

Boron
An important though often overlooked mineral that supports bone density. Found naturally in many plant foods: especially apples, pears,

potatoes, broccoli, parsley, soya and some nuts. Recommended daily intake about 3mg.

Calcium

Calcium is essential for healthy bones and proper nerve and muscle function. Found in sesame and other seeds, nuts, dark green leafy vegetables, soya, dairy produce and sardines. Standard advice from the menopause onwards is to have between 1000 and 1500mg a day in the diet, rather than as a supplement (50g of tofu contains about 650 mg of calcium). Daily intake should not exceed 2000mg.

Magnesium

An important mineral during the menopause as it can help to reduce hot flushing and tiredness. Magnesium may also help to maintain bone density. Found in green leafy vegetables, wholegrains, beans including soya, nuts, seeds and molasses. Best sourced by eating these foods as part of a balanced diet – recommended intake 750mg a day.

Zinc

Zinc is especially needed by reproductive tissue and the eyes. Found in seeds, especially pumpkin seeds and shellfish – oysters have very high levels! The recommended daily intake is 15mg.

Omega-3 oils

Polyunsaturated oils that are in high demand in nerve and reproductive tissue. Deficiency is common as these oils are found principally in oily fish and linseed. Deficiency is associated with depression. Ideally, intake of omega-3 and omega-6 oils should be linked – 1 part omega-3 oils to 3 parts omega-6 oils. Linseed is the best plant source – see herb profile.

Omega-6 oils

These oils are more commonly found in the western diet and deficiency is less common as a result. Evening Primrose and Borage oils are good sources and can help relieve breast tenderness and other pre-menstrual problems. Found in all seeds, virgin seed oils and nuts.

Natural supplements

There are a whole range of readily available 'super-foods', much cheaper than vitamin and mineral tablets and much better absorbed. They provide good nutrition though you may need to eat a lot to take in the same quantity as a vitamin/mineral supplement. Many on this list also contain appreciable levels of phytoestrogens.

- *Beansprouts* cleansing and nourishing, contain many minerals; alfa-alfa contains high levels of phytoestrogens (isoflavones) along with vitamins A, C and E
- *Lemon juice* drink juice of freshly squeezed lemon each morning with warm water (add honey if wanted); rich in vitamin C and bioflavonoids, aids liver detoxification
- *Linseed* sprinkle 1 tablespoon ground linseed on muesli or cereal each morning to encourage regular bowel movements; a major source of phytoestrogens and omega-3 oils
- *Molasses* an inexpensive natural supplement rich in minerals, especially iron, and vitamins B_6 and E
- *Oats* an excellent food and medicine: eat at breakfast to stabilise blood sugar levels, balance blood fat levels, reduce food cravings; helps strengthen nervous function (B vitamin and calcium content), good for nervous exhaustion, chronic stress and depression; improves stamina and can help with lowered libido
- *Parsley* a tonic and cleansing herb, good for arthritis and with good levels of vitamin C and E, iron, boron and phytoestrogens
- *Seaweed* harvested from the shore, seaweeds are mineral-rich – particularly iodine and calcium
- *Seeds* make a good snack: all contain significant levels of phytoestrogens, omega-6 oils and minerals such as iron and calcium; some such as pumpkin are rich in zinc
- *Soya, beans and lentils* all rich in phytoestrogens and omega-3 and -6 oils, soya contains useful levels of boron and calcium
- *Spirulina* a natural vitamin and mineral supplement in its own right, contains large amounts of B vitamins including B_{12} and like seaweed, a wide range of minerals

- *Tahini*   ground sesame seeds, very easy to use in cooking and on bread, rich in omega-6 oils and minerals, especially calcium
- *Wheatgerm*   contains large amounts of vitamin E, an important nutrient for helping with hot flushing.

Exercise

Every self-help book rightly lists exercise as one of the key things you can do to help yourself stay healthy, and this is just as much the case at the menopause. Exercise improves blood flow and circulation to organs and tissues throughout the body, strengthens muscles and ligaments, aids posture, increases alertness and well-being, helps control weight . . . in short, we humans were designed to exercise.

If you've got your exercise regime worked out and you really do make the most of your gym membership, you should probably skip this section. But what do you do if you are one of life's instinctive couch potatoes?

Firstly, **keeping active counts** – whether its walking to work, doing housework, gardening or playing with children. Simply using your body at work and at rest in a healthy non-stressed way maintains muscle tone and bulk. Increasing this type of activity can be one of the easiest ways to exercise more – getting off the bus a stop early, for example – and it should *not* be devalued just because it's a part of everyday life.

Secondly, **what kind of exercise do you enjoy**? Salsa dancing does not come high up most peoples list of aerobic exercise but not only is it good quality exercise, it's sociable and an enjoyable way to work out. Another good form of exercise that is particularly good for women with menstrual problems is Egyptian or belly dancing. It is equally valuable from the menopause onwards. This is one of the very best forms of exercise for the abdomen, lower back and pelvis. Improving blood flow to the pelvis – an area prone to congestion and pooling of blood, and containing the bladder, womb, vagina and rectum – can make a big difference. Better blood flow means better nutrition, and more exercise means better muscle and ligament tone. Put simply, these organs will stay in better shape and the chances of developing a range of problems including vaginal dryness, prolapsed bowel or womb, urinary incontinence or constipation will be much reduced. If dancing does not appeal to you, find some form of exercise that would be practicable for you to get to and might prove pleasurable. What about swimming, badminton, fencing, hill-walking and so on – all best done as a social as well as a physical exercise?

Lastly, **allow yourself time for relaxing exercise**. There are by now so many different forms of toning, relaxing exercise to choose from - from Alexander technique to yoga – that one is spoilt for choice. Learning even a little from one of these systems gives you the wherewithal to stretch and literally shake off the accumulated stress and tension that otherwise will stay clinging to your body and mind through the day. Although it may make you aware of muscles that you never knew you had, managing to do something like yoga or T'ai Chi each morning or evening brings unexpected benefits, not least a clearer mind and a more focused spirit. No one says its easy but it can make a big difference to one's quality of life.

Keeping a positive attitude

People talk about a 'positive attitude' as looking on the bright side of life, and seeing the half-drunk glass on the table, as half-full rather than half-empty. The glass is of course half-full! In the same way, in mid-life one can focus on life that has gone . . . or on life yet to be lived. Affirming your life till now, and all the positive ways it has unfolded is important, but as everyone knows, dwelling on the past prevents one from living in the present.

There is little space here to give more than a few hints about how to focus on the positive and connect with that part of you that manages to enjoy life and get things done. A good starting point is to quieten the 'voices' in one's mind that put one down and undermine self-confidence and self-esteem. Quietening these negative voices through keeping calm, focused and relaxed in the face of stress and tension is often the key to overcoming anxiety, and is certainly the simplest way to gain more out of life. However hard it may seem, even in the midst of emotional turmoil, it *is* possible to reduce the destructive effects of anxiety and stress and to develop a greater sense of self-control. Change does not necessarily come quickly but with persistence it does happen.

Many of the activities that help relieve anxiety and stress are well known and easy to do, especially within a group. Many will be equally helpful where lowered mood and depression are the main problem. Deep breathing exercises, visualisation, relaxation techniques, meditation, playing music, painting and drawing, relaxing and toning exercise – all help to nurture a deeper connection with the healing, strengthening, enlivening side to life that all too often gets little space in our time-pressured lives.

However much we may not be able to see it, and may feel surrounded and hemmed in by invincible walls, there is always a door that opens out into a freer world. Whether it is the power of the imagination, of visualisation, that takes you to a beautiful, protected place on a beach or in the mountains, or the tonic effect of regular relaxed exercise – fear, worry and anger can be healed.

Perhaps, in the last instance what is meant by cultivating a positive attitude is something close to this ancient prayer:

> God grant me the serenity
> To accept the things I cannot change
> The courage to change the things I can
> And the wisdom to know the difference.

5 | Using herbal medicines effectively

Over the last 10 years, people's understanding and use of herbal medicine has grown considerably with several herbs – notably St. John's Wort and Ginkgo – becoming some of the most commonly taken medicines of all. However, herbal medicine is quite complex and a little thought can go a long way towards maximising your chances of using herbs safely and effectively.

There are a number of things that anyone planning to use over the counter herbs should ask themselves before making a purchase:

- *What am I trying to treat?*
  This may sound like a silly question – but are you trying to treat a specific symptom, treat or prevent an underlying long-term problem, or simply improve health and vitality: herbs can be used on all three levels. Thinking in terms of the menopause, herbal remedies can be taken to relieve specific symptoms such as hot flushing, to prevent the development of menopausal problems as a whole or to improve a sense of well-being.

- *What herb(s) should I use?*
  The herb(s) you choose should correspond with your reason for taking them. If relieving hot flushes is the main aim then go for herbs such as Black Cohosh that act quickly. Taking foods/herbs such as Linseed or Fenugreek may lead to disappointment if you are expecting *instant* relief of symptoms, as both work to improve hormonal balance in the *medium to long term*. Likewise, St. John's Wort probably has no direct *hormonal* effect in treating menopausal problems, though as it raises mood and vitality it has much to offer in terms of improving quality of life. For simple relief of symptoms taking one single herb is often the best idea. Where you are trying to treat different problems at the same time or to combine the benefits of individual herbs, take up to a maximum of three herbs together. Recommended combinations are given at the end of each herb profile.

- *What is the best way to take them?*
It is very hard to generalise about the advantages and disadvantages of different types of herbal preparation. The quality of the herbs used to make the particular product is often as important as how the herbs have been processed. Advice about buying herbal remedies over the counter is found in the section below. Hot infusions are not a sensible way to take herbs for hot flushing – if you want to take an infusion allow it to cool first. Tinctures are most convenient if you want to combine a number of herbs – simply pour the appropriate amount of each herb together – though they do contain alcohol, which is 'heating' and unhelpful in hot flushing. Capsules and tablets can be the most convenient method of taking herbs. Capsules usually contain the powdered herb without additives though you may need to take several per dose. Tablets can contain a number of additives along with the herbal extract but you will probably need to swallow only one or two a day. Look for products that are 'pharmacopoeia standard' or 'standardised extracts', both of which should have been put through rigorous quality control checks.

- *What should I expect from treatment?*
Another very difficult question to answer! Typically, people notice improvements in their sense of well-being more quickly than relief of symptoms, though this is very variable. Improvement can set in with the first dose but more commonly signs of symptom relief take 1-2 weeks to occur, and can take up to 8-12 weeks to reach maximum effect. Of course, not everyone experiences improvement. When no change occurs this is for one of three reasons: for some reason in your case the herb is not effective; or the wrong herb has been chosen; or the herb is of poor quality. If you have tried a single herb without success, it may be worth trying a different herb with similar indications. For example, if you have taken Black Cohosh without effect, try taking a Red Clover or Wild Yam product.

Other things that will increase the chances of the herbal medicine working safely and effectively:

- *Good quality* Follow the advice given in the section below, when purchasing herbal products over the counter. Always check the sell-by date.

- *Compliance*   Taking herbal medicines as instructed means they will have a better chance of working effectively. Normally it is best to take herbs at regular times each day, and about 30 minutes before meals.

- *Interactions*   Some herbs, e.g. St. John's Wort interact with prescription medicines. If you are taking medicines prescribed by your doctor, discuss taking herbal medicines with your doctor or medical herbalist before starting treatment.

Buying herbal medicines over the counter

What should you look out for when buying herbal medicines? The following simple guidelines should help to ensure that you buy reasonable quality herbal medicines. Do not be tempted by extremely cheap herbal products – they are likely to be poor quality. It is usually more convenient to buy pre-packed capsules, tablets, essential oils and tinctures and to make up infusions and decoctions yourself (see next section for how to make).

- Buy from a reputable herb store that is knowledgeable about herbal medicines – you should be given clear, sensible information about what herbs might help and how to take them.

- Do not be afraid to ask what training assistants have had when they give you advice – if you receive a cold response to your question, shop elsewhere!

- Only buy mail order from established herbal suppliers.

- Buy organic herbs/products where available, or pharmacopoeia standard herbs, which have been properly tested to ensure that they contain only very low levels of pesticides and have not been subject to irradiation.

Buying dried herbs:

- Herbs lose their colour as they age – look for bright material that has been well dried and stored.

- Don't buy herbs that are in clear glass jars (unless kept in the dark), and don't buy herbal products that have been on display in the window.

- Good-quality aromatic herbs should have a distinct scent and taste.

Buying herbal products – capsules, tablets, etc.:
- Read the label – it should:
  - Name all constituents in the product
  - State the recommended daily dosage
  - State the weight of each capsule or tablet, or volume of bottle
  - List the weight of each constituent in a capsule, tablet, etc.
  - List the ratio of herb in the product (e.g. 1:3 = 1 part herb to 3 parts liquid)
- If it does not provide this information do not buy it.
- 'Pharmacopoeia-standard' herbs have met strict quality control standards and have not been concentrated or processed. They are therefore closer to their natural state than 'standardised extracts'. Standardised extracts should also have met strict quality control standards and have been concentrated so that smaller amounts of extracts need to be taken each day.

Making up herbal remedies

Infusions
Making an infusion is no more difficult than making a cup of tea.
- To make Sage tea, for example, use 1 level tsp of dried chopped leaf or 1 heaped tsp of fresh chopped leaf per cup. Put in a teapot and cover with a cupful of boiling water. Stir and leave to stand for 5-10 minutes. Strain and add a little honey if wanted. Allow to cool until lukewarm if taking an infusion for hot flushes. Dose 1-2 cups a day as required.

These measurements can be used to make infusions of leaves, flowers and chopped whole herb. Many herbs, e.g. Red Clover flowers, can be drunk at higher dosage: use 1 heaped tsp of dried chopped herb per cup and drink up to 4 or 5 cups a day.

Decoctions
Decoctions involve boiling tougher parts of herbs - roots, bark, berries - for about 20 minutes, as leaves and other more tender plant parts are often destroyed by boiling.

- To make a decoction of Chinese Angelica take 15g of chopped or sliced dried root and simmer in a non-aluminium saucepan with ¾ litre of water. Allow the water to evaporate until after about 20 minutes approx. ½ litre of water is left. Divide into 3-5 doses and store in a fridge. Decoctions will keep for up to 48 hours in a fridge.

These measurements can be used for other decoctions, though some herbs need to be taken at much lower levels. The standard dose for Black Cohosh is 200mg a day and is very difficult to decoct – better to take a capsule or tablet! Check the dosage for each herb, given at the end of each profile.

Agnus Castus ~ *Vitex agnus castus*

Key uses: irregular menstrual cycle, menstrual and hormonally-related headaches; hormonal imbalance at the menopause; pre-menstrual problems: period pains, breast tenderness, fluid retention and acne; infertility; polycystic ovaries; to increase breast milk production.

Uses during menopause: Often growing close to the Mediterranean sea, Agnus castus's use for menstrual and menopausal problems dates back 1,000's of years. The small round berries support progesterogenic activity and promote hormonal balance throughout the menstrual cycle. As a result Agnus castus is often useful in the months and years before the menopause (peri-menopause), when menstrual irregularity and heavy bleeding can be real problems. Agnus castus can help to re-establish a regular cycle and relieve menstrually-related problems such as period pains, breast tenderness, migraine, headaches and acne. With Lady's Mantle, it makes a good treatment for heavy menstrual bleeding and flooding. In view of the berries' subtle effects on hormonal balance, Agnus castus should be seen as a general treatment for menopausal symptoms, perhaps even as part of an alternative to HRT, and can be taken long term to aid adaptation to lowered oestrogen and progesterone levels. In this case, it should be combined with Black Cohosh.

Other traditional uses: The positive hormonal influence that Agnus castus exerts on the menstrual cycle, ovaries and womb makes it a key herb for treating infertility. In situations where impaired fertility is due to hormonal imbalance e.g. polycystic ovary disease, the herb can directly increase fertility and re-establish regular ovulation. The berries stimulate breast milk secretion and have a long traditional use for this purpose. Having anti-androgenic activity the herb is useful wherever excess androgens are causing hormonal disturbance, e.g. in acne occurring pre-menstrually and in polycystic ovarian syndrome. Medical herbalists also prescribe it for conditions such as endometriosis and fibroids.

Research: Research into Agnus castus' hormonal activity has been underway for over 30 years, and despite some mixed results, there can be little doubt that some women benefit greatly from taking the berries or extract, especially for pre-menstrual problems. Agnus castus is thought to act on the hypothalamus and pituitary gland (situated at the base of the brain), influencing release of several hormones, especially those that control progesterone release by the ovaries. It has progesterogenic and anti-androgenic activity. There is so far little research into Agnus castus' use for menopausal problems but both the progesterogenic action, and the herb's ability to encourage a regular menstrual cycle, indicate that traditional use for menstrual irregularity close to the menopause – and for hormonal balance thereafter – is well founded.

Cautions: Nausea is an occasional side-effect. Not advisable to take at the same time as other hormonal treatment e.g. HRT, the contraceptive pill or IVF.

Dosage: Berries
Berries/powder   – 0.5-1g a day
Capsule   – 0.5-1g a day (1-2 capsules)
Tablet   – as recommended by manufacturer
Fluid Extract (1:1) – up to 20 drops a day
Tincture (1:5)   – up to 5ml a day
All best taken as a single dose on waking in the morning, when the pituitary gland is most active.

Combinations:
With Black Cohosh to promote hormonal balance and for hormonally-related headaches
With Lady's Mantle for irregular menstruation and to reduce heavy menstrual bleeding
With Chinese Angelica as a hormonal tonic

Black Cohosh ~ *Cimicifuga racemosa*

Key uses: Menopausal problems; neuralgia; nervous tension; sleep problems; tinnitus (ringing in the ears); muscle pains and cramps; arthritis; cramps; pre-menstrual complaints and period pains; asthma.

Uses during menopause: One of the most valuable herbs for the menopause, Black Cohosh can sometimes halt symptoms entirely within a matter of days. Hot flushing, poor sleep and nervous irritability are key indications for this herb's use and its gently sedative activity means that it will help to take the edge off anxiety and tension headaches as well. A calming, centre-ing herb then, worth considering for most menopausal problems, it can at the same time reduce feelings of fluster and embarrassment commonly brought on by hot flushing, sweating and the rapid temperature changes that go with it. With significant anti-inflammatory activity, Black Cohosh is a key herb for inflammation affecting muscles and joints, and in my practice I prescribe it routinely for the type of osteoarthritis that develops in the wrists, hands or fingers (and sometimes feet) during the menopause. When combined with St. John's Wort, Black Cohosh also makes a valuable remedy for nervous exhaustion and depressed mood, the combination helping specifically during the menopause.

Other traditional uses: Black Cohosh has many traditional applications: for nerve pain and neurological disorders and can be used successfully in conditions such as tinnitus, dizziness and vertigo. It combines well with Feverfew for chronic headache and migraine. For muscle pain, inflammatory arthritis and rheumatic conditions (especially when associated with hormonal change), it can sometimes prove dramatically effective, relieving symptoms and reversing the course of the illness. As an antispasmodic, it helps to ease cramps and restless muscles, making it potentially useful for 'restless legs'. It is commonly taken to relieve pre-menstrual problems, especially period pains and headaches. Having a sedative and relaxing effect on the body it tends to lower raised blood pressure; and as an expectorant may be used in whooping cough and asthma. Traditional native American use (the herb comes from the east coast of the USA) includes fevers and feverish conditions, such as influenza and measles.

Research: Since the 1950's, research into Black Cohosh's usefulness in menopausal symptoms has been underway in Germany. Extracts of the herb have been shown repeatedly to have distinct benefit, relieving hot flushing, sweating, sleep disturbances and depressive moods. In 1998, an analysis of 8 clinical trials concluded that Black Cohosh extract might be a safe and effective alternative to HRT, where HRT was contraindicated or its use rejected. Other clinical research has reached the same conclusion. In one clinical trial, also published in 1998, improvement in symptoms occurred within two weeks and after 6 months approx. 90% of the women taking the extract had experienced symptom reduction. There is also the suggestion – not as yet researched in detail – that Black Cohosh may inhibit mineral loss (calcium) from bone and thus have protective activity against osteoporosis in menopausal women. Curiously, Black Cohosh does not, as previously thought, have significant oestrogenic activity.

Cautions: Indigestion is an occasional side effect.

Dosage: 40-200 mg of herb a day:
Dried root (decoction)   – up to 200mg a day
Capsule/powder   – up to 200mg a day
Tincture (1:10)   – 0.4-2ml a day
Fluid extract (1:1)   – 0.2ml a day (4 drops)

Combinations:
With Wild Yam and/or Agnus Castus for hot flushing and to promote hormonal balance
With Wild Yam and/or Devil's Claw for inflammatory arthritis
With St. John's Wort for menopausal exhaustion and depression
With Ginkgo for tinnitus
With Scullcap or Vervain for tension headaches and anxiety

Chinese Angelica (Dong Quai) ~ *Angelica sinensis*

Key uses: Menopause – as a tonic; circulatory problems including arteriosclerosis; irregular menstruation; period pains; infertility; chronic hepatitis.

Uses during menopause: Taken on a daily basis by millions of Asian women, Dong Quai is the principal women's tonic in traditional Chinese medicine. With a warming and pleasant flavour it stimulates digestion, blood flow and vitality, and is thought to have a tonic effect on the womb and reproductive system as a whole. During the menopause, it is clearly helpful in raising energy levels where deficient, and it finds specific use in increasing blood flow to congested or cold, poorly served areas of the body – the pelvis, hands and feet, for example. It is unlikely to reduce symptoms such as hot flushing (see *Research* below) but may well improve vaginal tone and promote a sense of well being – and in this way has been considered to have aphrodisiac properties in the past.

Other traditional uses: Dong Quai is often taken to relieve menstrual problems, especially period pains and an irregular cycle. It needs to be taken cautiously where menstrual bleeding is heavy but will help the body to 'build' blood, especially in iron-deficiency anaemia – and is seen first and foremost as a 'blood tonic' in traditional Chinese medicine. It has a major effect on the circulation, keeping the blood thin, reducing arteriosclerosis and improving circulation to the periphery – head, hands and feet. Dong Quai has a protective action on the heart, supports a regular heart beat, and is often prescribed by practitioners for angina. It also protects the liver from damage and stimulates liver metabolism. As a mildly pungent, hot remedy it stimulates digestion and relieves wind. As these last indications suggest, Dong Quai may be useful for both women and men.

Research: There is little evidence to show that Dong Quai has a direct effect on menopausal symptoms such as hot flushing or lowered mood. In fact, the only clinical trial to date to investigate Dong Quai's value in treating menopausal symptoms found it to have no more effect than placebo. Furthermore, contrary to expectation, Dong Quai appears not to have oestrogenic activity, so its ability to act hormonally and influence the reproductive organs is being questioned. Despite this, Dong Quai is still likely to have value during the menopause and after, if for no other reason than its powerful tonic effects on the heart and circulation (see above): improved cardio-vascular function leads to better tissue health and overall vitality, especially where blood flow is weak or congested. Although Dong Quai's role in treating chronic liver problems is not substantiated as yet, there is evidence that the root stimulates liver metabolism, increasing the organ's capacity to clear toxins from the body, and promoting liver health as a consequence.

Cautions: avoid – if taking prescribed medicines such as warfarin or heparin (anti-coagulants); during acute viral infections; tendency to bleed easily – *including heavy menstrual bleeding.*

Dosage: root
Decoction/in food – up to 10g a day
Capsule/powder   – up to 5g a day
Tincture (1:3)   – up to 15ml a day

Combinations:
With Agnus castus and Fenugreek or Wild Yam for vaginal dryness and reduced libido
With Ginger for wind and digestive weakness
With Ginkgo for poor peripheral circulation

Cranberry ~ *Vaccinium macrocarpon*

Key uses: Cystitis and urethritis, bladder irritation, thrush.

Uses at the menopause: An excellent remedy for urinary tract infections, Cranberry can be successfully used to both treat and prevent problems such as cystitis and urethritis. Chronic infection or irritation, including thrush, bladder irritability and frequency, are quite common from the menopause onwards and Cranberries make a first rate medicine for such problems – safe and effective, even when taken long-term. For best results, brave the very sour taste and drink the unsweetened juice or take Cranberry extract, either way Cranberry will help to disinfect the urinary tubules and make it less likely that you will need to rely on antibiotic treatment for chronic urinary infections. Taken at the first signs of infection, Cranberry can prevent the onset of acute cystitis, though in such situations it is generally best combined with herbs such as Kava or Echinacea and, of course, lots of water. Cranberry may also be used long term to prevent the development of calcium carbonate kidney stones and has a reputation for helping in late onset diabetes .

Research: Research published in the *Journal of the American Medical Association* in 1994 found that Cranberry juice reduced the need for antibiotics in women suffering from chronic urinary tract infection. It seems likely that Cranberry works by making it more difficult for bacteria to cling to the urinary tract wall, and infection is therefore more easily flushed out. It is possible that the same effect occurs in the digestive tract and Cranberry may also help to prevent gastro-intestinal infections. Like its close relative, Bilberry (Vaccinium myrtillus) Cranberry is powerfully anti-oxidant and supports a healthy circulation.

Cautions: Do not take in kidney infections or other kidney disease.

Dosage: Berries or juice
Juice   – up to 500ml a day
Capsule/tablet – as recommended by manufacturer

Combinations:
With Kava for irritable bladder and urinary frequency
With Echinacea and/or Grapefruit seed extract for acute cystitis

Fenugreek ~ *Trigonella foenum-graecum*

Key uses: Indigestion and gastritis; menopausal symptoms including hot flushing and vaginal dryness; irritable bowel including diarrhoea and constipation; convalescence; raised blood fats; late onset diabetes; bronchitis.

Uses during menopause: A strongly flavoured herb, Fenugreek seeds are useful in helping to support oestrogen levels within the body during the menopause and on into later life. Fenugreek is probably most useful in helping to reduce or prevent vaginal dryness, soreness and inflammation, as well as dry skin in general. The seeds should be eaten as food and a lotion can be applied locally to the vagina or the skin as required. The seeds have a longstanding reputation as an aphrodisiac and given their oestrogenic action may well help to improve libido and support sexual activity. The seeds can be taken to relieve hot flushing. Fenugreek may also have a role in preventing cardio-vascular disease from the menopause onwards – as well as being oestrogenic the seeds lower cholesterol levels. Lastly, Fenugreek's established oestrogenic activity has led to its use as a paste applied to the breasts to encourage breast enlargement. It appears to be effective – offering a cheap and safe alternative to silicon implants!

Other traditional uses: As a food: Fenugreek is a concentrated food, providing high levels of protein, good quality oils, and a range of vitamins and minerals comparable to Linseed. As a result it makes a good remedy for convalescence and debilitated states, and to promote weight gain in anorexia (one problem with it is that it can encourage unwanted weight gain). As a medicine, it soothes and heals sore, inflamed or ulcerated tissue throughout the digestive tract, and can be used to treat conditions as diverse as mouth ulcers, gastritis and irritable bowel; it also soothes hot, dry, sore throats, chesty coughs and bronchitis. Fenugreek is a herb/food to include when treating raised cholesterol levels as well as the cardio-vascular problems that follow from disordered fat metabolism. Likewise, it can prove valuable as part of a comprehensive approach to treating late onset diabetes. Applied to the skin, a lotion or poultice promotes wound and burn healing, eases the pain of sores and tumours, and 'draws' boils.

Research: Research over the past 10 years has shown that Fenugreek seeds have surprising potential as a medicine. The seeds are strongly oestrogenic and can be valuable in menopausal symptoms such as hot flushing and vaginal dryness. Several clinical trials have also shown that the seeds are effective in lowering levels of 'bad' fats within the blood – cholesterol, LDL, VLDL and triglycerides, while leaving levels of the 'good' HDL unchanged. It is important to stress however that people in these trials took very large quantities of the defatted seeds – 100g a day, way above normal dietary intake. In a number of clinical trials, diabetic patients who took between 15 and 100g of the seeds a day had significantly improved blood sugar control.

Cautions: none known.

Dosage:
Seeds (crushed/ground) – up to a 1–2 cupfuls a day
Decoction/lotion   – up to 30g a day: simmer in water for 5
                       minutes, strain
Capsule   – normally up to 5g a day
Tincture (1:3)   – up 15ml a day
                       (less effective than other preparations)
Poultice   – place seeds (preferably ground) in cloth,
                       soak in boiling water for 5 minutes, when
                       sufficiently cooled secure on affected area

Combinations:
With Agnus Castus and Chinese Angelica for vaginal dryness and increasing libido
With Turmeric for raised blood cholesterol levels

Hops ~ *Humulus lupulus*

Key uses: poor sleep; anxiety; headache; poor appetite.

Uses during menopause: Not one of the most commonly taken herbs for the menopause, hops – as found in beer – are strongly oestrogenic, and women hop-pickers often experience menstrual irregularity during the harvesting season as a result of daily exposure. Hop 'flowers' rarely figure on their own in a herbal approach to the menopause but where there is weak digestion, stomach cramps, wind and bloating, poor appetite or digestive-type headaches, hops can in small quantities be a good friend – it's distinctive, strong aroma and taste stimulating digestive activity and improving absorption of nutrients, and even in beer, hops will tend to work in this way. Hops also makes a good sedative and it is here that the herb may prove of most use during the menopause. Combined with herbs such as Kava Kava and Scullcap, Hops will reduce excitability and encourage better sleep, easing the 'spinning head' and anxiety that keep one lying wide awake in bed into the small hours. A Hop-stuffed pillow can also be helpful. In short, Hops' oestrogenic activity makes it a herb to consider whenever a bitter digestive or sedative remedy is called for, though as indicated below (Safety) it should *not* be taken in depressed states or nervous exhaustion.

Research: Though a poorly researched remedy, there is plenty of evidence that Hops works as a sedative and digestive stimulant, different studies showing that it promotes sleep and increases gastric secretions. The herb's oestrogenic activity has not been fully established, though empirical evidence clearly indicates such an effect.

Dosage:
Infusion (dried strobiles) – up to 1g a day
Capsule   – up to 1g a day
Tincture (1:5)   – up to 3ml a day

Safety: Avoid in depression/depressed mood.

Combinations:
With Kava Kava and/or Scullcap for sleep disturbance, headache and anxiety (though not when linked with depression)
With Liquorice and Chamomile for poor appetite, weak digestion, wind and bloating

Kava Kava ~ *Piper methysticum*

Key uses: Anxiety and stress-related symptoms; poor sleep; chronic or recurrent cystitis.

Uses during menopause: Kava has a lot to offer as a safe, natural *and* effective treatment for anxiety, low spirits and stress-related symptoms. Of course, Kava cannot treat the factors giving rise to stress but it can help to reduce responses to them – a calmer, more relaxed feeling, better quality sleep and a chance to take a step back from the stress and regain focus. There are also indications that Kava improves concentration – perhaps by reducing stress-levels. Kava is an effective remedy for muscle spasm and will help to relax tense shoulders and muscle cramps. Kava is also a useful urinary antiseptic that can be used to treat chronic or recurrent urinary tract infections.

Research: Kava's ability to calm and relax has been validated in a number of clinical trials. In one German clinical trial (1991), 40 women with menopausal symptoms took Kava standardised extract (containing 210mg kava lactones) or placebo for 8 weeks. The results showed a significant reduction in symptoms of anxiety and depression and an increase in sense of well-being. Other menopausal symptoms such as hot flushing and sleep disturbance also improved. Unusually, while Kava improves sleep it is only mildly sedative, so there is little risk of drowsiness on waking, as can happen with herbs such as Valerian.

Dosage: Dried root
Decoction   – up to 3g a day
Capsule   – up to 3g a day
Standardised extracts – up to 200mg kava lactones per day

Safety: At normal doses Kava rarely produces side-effects. Excessive doses can cause skin rashes.

Combinations:
With St. John's Wort for depression and nervous exhaustion
With Scullcap and/or Valerian for anxiety, panic attacks and insomnia
With Black Cohosh for headaches and dizziness

Korean Ginseng ~ *Panax ginseng*

Key uses: Exhaustion, depleted states and convalescence; long-term stress; preparation for stressful events e.g. exams, physically demanding events.

Uses during menopause: Despite its use for over 5,000 years as a male tonic and aphrodisiac, Ginseng has much to recommend its use during the menopause and indeed later in life too. In traditional Chinese medicine, Ginseng tones *Qi* (energy), calms the spirit and strengthens *Yin* where deficient, all valuable effects in states of depletion and chronic tiredness. In western terms, the herb is an 'adaptogen', increasing the body and mind's ability to adapt to and cope with stress of all kinds. Ginseng can therefore be taken to promote physical endurance and resistance to the cold, to increase mental capacity under stress and, given its anti-ageing activity, to tone and improve stamina in the frail and elderly. Add in the root's potential to aid in situations as varied as prolapsed organs, late onset diabetes and heart disease and one can to see that Ginseng has much to offer. During the menopause Ginseng can be taken specifically to improve vitality and relieve exhaustion, and may help to reduce excessive sweating. As a stimulant herb however, it is best avoided in anxiety, tension and poor sleep. Except during convalescence and in the elderly, Ginseng is normally taken for about 6-10 weeks at a time, with a gap in treatment before starting another course. Caffeine tends to undercut Ginseng's strengthening activity, and caffeine drinks, etc. should be avoided when taking the root.

Research: One of the most intensively researched herbs, Ginseng has an undoubted ability to support health and vitality when the body is under stress. Partly it achieves this by supporting adrenal gland function, which is often depleted by long term stress. Ginseng may also have a direct hormonal benefit during the menopause as it contains a number of oestrogenic-type constituents. It helps to prevent degenerative disease, including certain types of heart disease and cancer, though it should not be taken to prevent or treat cancers such as breast or cervical cancer.

Cautions: Do not take during acute illness or in high blood pressure. If taking prescribed medicines, especially anti-coagulants, consult your doctor or herbalist before taking Ginseng.

Dosage: dried root
Capsule or powder – 0.5-3g a day
(start with 0.5g and increase if required)
Tablet   – As recommended by manufacturer

Combinations:
With St. John's Wort for nervous exhaustion
With Black Cohosh for tiredness and hot flushing

Lady's Mantle ~ *Alchemilla vulgaris*

Key uses: Irregular menstrual cycle; heavy or intermenstrual bleeding.

Uses during menopause: A valuable herb if menstrual irregularities occur close to the menopause, Lady's Mantle is regarded as a specific for heavy menstrual bleeding. The leaves are markedly astringent and traditionally taken to staunch and heal wounds. This same styptic property can make an infusion of the herb effective in controlling flooding and profuse menstrual bleeding, especially where clotting is present as well. There is the suggestion that the herb may have a progesterogenic action and help to promote a regular menstrual cycle. Taken on its own or with Agnus Castus, Lady's Mantle is a herb of choice for painful and irregular periods, and is commonly prescribed by medical herbalists to treat conditions such as endometriosis and fibroids. In view of its possible hormonal activity, Lady's Mantle is now being used during the menopause as well, helping the body to adjust and adapt to changed hormone levels. The herb is traditionally thought to improve digestion and liver function acting as a decongestant. The most unusual traditional use is recorded by the English herbalist, John Gerard (1597): Lady's Mantle is reputed to tone and strengthen the breasts and "when they be too great or flaggie, it maketh them lesser and harder". Gerard had a knack of getting things right, so it could be worth a try.

Research: There has been little research into the herb, though recent research in Russia found that Lady's Mantle reduces blood viscosity.

Cautions: A safe herb with no known side-effects or interactions.

Dosage: dried leaf
Infusion   – up to 10g a day (1 heaped teaspoonful per cup: infuse for 10-15 minutes)
Capsule and powder – up to 5g a day
Tincture (1:5)   – up to 20ml a day

Combinations:
With Agnus castus for heavy menstrual bleeding, irregular menstrual cycle and period pains

Linseed (or Flaxseed) ~ *Linum usitatissimum*

Key uses: phytoestrogenic aid for the menopause; nutrient; constipation and bowel disorders.

Uses during menopause: Linseed's botanical name means 'most useful' and for such a little known plant, the seeds have a remarkable range of uses. They make an effective bulk laxative, especially valuable in chronic constipation and irritable bowel syndrome – take with about 5 times their volume of water. More significantly, the seeds are phytoestrogen-rich and ground Linseed makes an excellent dietary supplement during the menopause, supporting oestrogen levels and hormonal adaptation. Furthermore, Linseed contains very high levels of omega-3 polyunsaturated fatty acids and has distinct cancer preventative activity. For these therapeutic benefits, it is essential to grind the seed before eating – unground seeds make a good bulk laxative but all the nutritional goodness goes straight through! Once ground the seeds must be stored in a cool refrigerator or they will rapidly go rancid.

Research: Linseed has unusually high levels of α-linolenic acid, an omega-3 polyunsaturated fatty acid, similar to those found in fish oils. Omega-3 oils influence many different factors within the body, all having a protective activity on the heart and circulation, and helping to reduce heart irregularities. There is evidence too that they confer a protective activity against cancer, and ground Linseed appears to have specific protective activity against endometrial and breast cancer: it is rich in omega-3 oils, which are deficient in most western diets, in phytoestrogens which are thought to reduce the impact of estradiol, and in mucilage and fibre, which prevents reabsorption of unwanted oestrogens from the intestines.

Cautions: Take plenty of water with Linseed. Keep ground seed in airtight container in a refrigerator.

Dosage: Seed
Ground seed   – up to 25g a day – about 1 heaped tbsp
Oil (cold-pressed and refrigerated) – up to 25ml a day (1 tbsp)

Combinations:
With ground Fenugreek seed as a dietary supplement for the menopause

Liquorice ~ *Glycyrrhiza glabra*

Key uses: Tonic for the menopause, menopausal symptoms such as hot flushing; chronic inflammatory problems including some types of arthritis; stomach problems including gastritis.

Uses during menopause: The same sticky black root that children like to chew is a powerful medicine, particularly good for chronic inflammation. Used by herbalists to treat conditions like asthma, stomach ulcers and rheumatoid arthritis, Liquorice makes a valuable contribution in many menopausal problems. Oestrogenic, liver protective, anti-inflammatory and a good all-round tonic, Liquorice root helps to strengthen and stimulate adrenal gland function – key organs in coping with stress and in re-establishing hormonal balance at the menopause. In Russia, Liquorice root tea was a common home remedy for menopausal symptoms such as hot flushing and poor vitality, its use going back several hundred years. In combination with other hormonally-active herbs it can provide effective relief for these and other problems, such as osteoarthritis, dry and itchy skin, chronic exhaustion and depression. If you are prone to fluid retention and puffiness, it should be used sparingly as in large doses it encourages fluid retention.

Research: A widely researched herb, Liquorice, and its constituents, were at one time the main conventional treatment for peptic ulcers. Its strong anti-inflammatory activity being similar to cortico-steroids, it can be taken to good effect in many chronic inflammatory illnesses. The root has anti-viral properties and stimulates interferon production – making it potentially useful in treating hepatitis. Its strong oestrogenic activity has been known for over 50 years.

Cautions: Do not take in high blood pressure, kidney disease or in pregnancy. If taking prescribed medicines, especially medication for the heart or cortico-steroids, consult your doctor or herbalist before taking Liquorice.

Dosage: dried root
Root (chewed)   – up to 3g a day
Capsule or powder – up to 2g a day
Tincture (1:5)   – up to 10ml a day

Combinations:
With Black Cohosh for many menopausal symptoms including hot flushing and chronic tiredness
With Scullcap and/or Kava for the effects of long term stress and anxiety
With Sage for excessive sweating, sore throats and as a wash for mouth ulcers

Motherwort ~ *Leonorus cardiaca*

Key uses: General tonic – particularly helpful in anxiety and nervous debility; palpitations and minor heart irregularities; pre-menstrual tension and period pains; poor appetite.

Uses during menopause: With its distinctly bitter taste, Motherwort stimulates appetite and digestion while exerting a relaxing effect on the nervous system. Combined with its stabilising activity on the heart – it's a good remedy for palpitations and heart irregularity – this makes the herb a useful tonic in nervous debility and exhaustion, long term anxiety and loss of appetite. Motherwort contains some phytoestrogenic compounds, though it is not clear how much they influence its overall activity. Given the herb's traditional use for pre-menstrual problems and as an aid in childbirth, it would be surprising if there was no beneficial hormonal activity to complement its tonic effects on the digestion, heart and nervous system. The 17th century English herbalist, Nicholas Culpeper, sums up Motherwort's virtues in characteristic fashion: "There is no better herb to drive away melancholy vapours from the heart, to strengthen it and make the mind cheerful, blithe and merry". Another old English saying suggests a more curmudgeonly approach: "Drink Motherwort tea and live to be a source of continuous astonishment and frustration to waiting heirs"!

Research: Limited clinical research in the west indicates that Motherwort, as its botanical name suggests, has a directly supportive activity on the heart, making it valuable in nervous heart conditions, arrhythmias, and the early stages of heart failure. Research into the very similar Chinese Motherwort (*L. heterophyllus*) indicates that the herb slows a rapid heartbeat, lowers blood pressure, aids the treatment of coronary heart disease, stimulates menstruation and has anti-cancer properties.

Cautions: Avoid in heavy menstrual bleeding; do not take during pregnancy.

Dosage: dried herb
Infusion   – 5g a day (or up to 15g a day for 3-4 days)
Capsule   – up to 3g a day
Tincture (1:5) – up to 15ml a day

Combinations:
With Dong Quai (Chinese Angelica) for palpitations and heart irregularity
With Sage as a general tonic during the menopause, and for loss of appetite

Red Clover ~ *Trifolium pratense*

Key uses: Phytoestrogenic – helpful in relieving hot flushing and other menopausal symptoms; swollen glands, acne and chronic skin problems including eczema and psoriasis.

Uses during menopause: Following research in Australia on Red Clover isoflavones, Red Clover has shot to fame as a herb for the menopause, and possible alternative to HRT. Though there is little evidence of the herb being used in the past during the menopause, the flowerheads contain high levels of isoflavones and are strongly oestrogenic. Red Clover therefore provides a useful route for balancing falling oestrogen levels, and given the herb's cleansing and detoxifying activity, there are other reasons why Red Clover – as an infusion, capsule or tincture – may be the herb of choice: chronic skin conditions, chronic constipation and a tendency to swollen glands or fluid retention can all benefit from it.

Red Clover *isoflavone* extract is well worth a try, if other herbal approaches, e.g. Black Cohosh and Agnus Castus, have failed to bring relief to menopausal symptoms. Long term use of Red Clover isoflavones may well be preferable to HRT, though a certain amount of caution is advised in taking such products, which do not have the longstanding traditional use that supports use of Red Clover as a herb.

Other traditional uses: Red Clover is a good detoxifier, typically used to support all kinds of congestion - lymphatic and glandular congestion, a sluggish liver and constipation, and the symptoms that accompany it e.g. skin problems, fluid retention, swollen glands. Often combined with other detoxifying herbs such as Marigold (*Calendual officinalis*) and Blue Flag (*Iris versicolor*), Red Clover is one of the most useful herbs for acne and eczema, proving of value in both children and adults. It can also be taken in combination with Cleavers (*Galium aparine*) to aid lymphatic drainage and clear fluid retention. Traditionally, Red Clover has been used in the treatment of cancer, in particular breast cancer, though the herb is best seen as having cancer-protective activity rather than as being a treatment for cancer.

Research: Though there can be no doubt that Red Clover has a marked oestrogenic activity, the precise way in which the herb works is not fully understood. The flowers contain up to 2.5% isoflavones, which are phytoestrogenic and appear to work in one of two ways depending on oestrogen levels within the body.

When *lowered*, for example at the menopause, the isoflavones are thought to complement the body's own oestrogen increasing overall levels and reducing symptoms of oestrogen deficiency. Several clinical trials in Australia have investigated the use of Red Clover extracts for menopausal problems but have not shown the extract to be effective. There are conflicting views on whether Red Clover, and isoflavones in general, help to protect the heart and circulation in post-menopausal women.

When *raised*, the isoflavones are thought to compete with the body's own circulating oestrogens for receptor sites. Being only weakly oestrogenic, when the isoflavones 'lock on' to oestrogen receptor sites the net effect is to reduce oestrogenic activity within the body. In particular, isoflavones may reduce levels of oestradiol, raised levels of which are associated with increased chances of developing breast cancer. *This is the theory* – it is not established fact. As a cancer preventative, Red Clover is best taken on professional advice; where breast cancer has been diagnosed Red Clover must *only* be taken on professional advice.

Cautions: Take *only* on professional advice in oestrogen-dependent cancers.

Dosage: Dried flowerheads
Infusion   – up to 10g a day
Capsule/powder – up to 5g a day
Tincture (1:5)   – up to 20ml a day
Tablets   – as recommended by the manufacturer

Combinations:
With Black Cohosh for long term relief of menopausal symptoms
With Echinacea and Agnus Castus for acne and skin problems related to menstruation or menopause
With Linseed and/or Liquorice for chronic constipation

Sage ~ *Salvia officinalis*

Key uses: General tonic – especially during the menopause; hot flushing, excessive sweating; stress and anxiety; sore throats, tonsillitis, mouth ulcers; weak digestion, loss of appetite, wind; healing wounds.

Uses during menopause: Sage makes an interesting, strongly flavoured tea with distinct benefit for menopausal symptoms. It is frequently taken to relieve hot flushing and excessive sweating, especially hormonally-related night sweats (drink *cold* rather than hot tea), and can prove quite effective in reducing symptoms. It has a wide range of other potential uses, including an ability to soothe anxious, irritable and mildly depressed nervous states. With a tonic activity on both the digestive and nervous systems, Sage is particularly valuable where the nervous system has been subject to long term stress. Like its close relative Rosemary, Sage may also improve memory. The 16th century English herbalist, William Turner (1551) noted that Sage "restores natural heat . . . comforts the vital spirits . . . helps the memory, and quickens the senses".

A useful recipe for making Sage tea: Use two level teaspoons of dried Sage leaf (heaped, if fresh leaf) in half a litre/one pint of boiling water, steep for an hour, drain. When cold take 1 tablespoon every hour or two until sweats are overcome.

Other traditional uses: Sage has powerful antiseptic, antioxidant and anti-inflammatory properties, a combination that lies behind its regular use as a gargle and mouthwash for sore throats, tonsillitis, hoarseness, mouth ulcers and gingivitis. Its hot, dry nature also makes it valuable for many catarrhal problems. As a digestive tonic it stimulates appetite and digestive secretions, and eases wind and bloating. Long term use strengthens the whole digestive process and improves absorption of nutrients. Sage also has the ability to speed up wound healing. One of the most prized of European medicinal plants, Sage has always been seen as a herb of longevity, promoting good health and vitality into old age. The ancient saying goes "Why should a man die while sage grows in the garden". The gender may be wrong – Sage has more to offer women than men – but the meaning, that Sage supports health and longevity is undoubtedly correct. Sage tea can also be used as a toning hair rinse which helps to keep dark hair from greying!

Research: The little research to date into Sage's medicinal value suggests that this is a herb with great potential. The herb's oestrogenic activity has been confirmed though the constituents responsible are yet to be identified. It's ability to reduce sweating has also been established though how this effect is achieved is not known. The herb's essential oil is powerfully antiseptic. Research in Newcastle (1998) indicates that Sage may have value in the treatment of Alzheimer's disease. Other research points to Sage having a relaxant, tranquilising effect on the mind.

Cautions: Do not take in high blood pressure, epilepsy and pregnancy. If taking prescribed medicines, consult your doctor or herbalist before taking Sage long-term.

Dosage: Dried herb
Infusion   – up to 3g a day – $^{1}/_{2}$ to 1 tsp per cup (also see above)
Capsule   – up to 1.5g a day
Tincture (1:5) – up to 7.5ml a day

Combinations:
With Black Cohosh for hot flushing and night sweats
With Motherwort as an all round tonic during the menopause
With Kava for anxiety and mood swings
With Echinacea for sore throats and mouth ulcers

St. John's Wort ~ *Hypericum perforatum*

Key uses: Mild to moderate depression, despondency, anxiety, panic, fear; related problems such as nervous exhaustion, insomnia, headaches; seasonal affective disorder; improves motivation, concentration and emotional stability; viral infections, including herpes sores and influenza.

Uses during menopause: St. John's Wort is a key herb for lowered mood, poor sleep and nervous exhaustion at any time in life, and there is a lot to commend its use around the time of the menopause. Disturbed and poor quality sleep almost inevitably undermines one's mood and self-confidence in the long term, and nervous exhaustion is itself a sign of vitality at a low ebb. St. John's Wort has the happy ability to raise the spirits and strengthen nervous function so that one can again find the resources to cope. Sleep quality is improved, the gloomy clouds of depression are lifted to some degree and a more stable emotional base means that life can be brought back under control once more. St. John's Wort will not relieve hormonally-based problems on its own and needs to be combined with herbs such as Black Cohosh to relieve symptoms such as hot flushing and night sweats. This combination can also prove valuable, perhaps with Devil's Claw, for osteoarthritis that flares up during the menopause.

Other traditional uses: St. John's Wort has been used as a medicine to treat depression and melancholy for at least 2,500 years. It also has anti-viral properties that make it potentially valuable in treating infections as varied as cold sores, 'flu and glandular fever. St. John's Wort is unlikely to be sufficient on its own in such situations, but viral infections often take root against a background of nervous exhaustion and depletion – states where St. John's Wort can be of significant use. St. John's Wort oil applied topically, and the flowers/herb taken internally, both encourage tissue repair, healing wounds – St. John's Wort used to be known as 'the military herb' in Spain, and controlling inflammation. St. John's Wort also has a longstanding reputation as a painkiller, helping to relieve nerve pain e.g. sciatica and toothache – again applied topically on the skin and/or taken internally.

Research: By now one of the most extensively researched herbal medicines of all, there is a large body of evidence confirming its value as an anti-depressant. In over 25 clinical trials St. John's Wort has been found to be as effective as conventional anti-depressants, but with a much better safety profile. In fact, in some clinical trials people taking St. John's Wort experienced fewer side effects than those taking placebo i.e. a medicinally inert substance! Besides being a safe and effective remedy for mild to moderate depression, research indicates that St. John's Wort can be effective in treating seasonal affective disorder (the winter blues), improving sleep quality and concentration, and physical performance in athletes. Add in a beneficial activity on the liver and evidence of a powerful ability to heal wounds and it is clear the St. John's Wort is much more than simply an anti-depressant.

Cautions: Safe in its own right, St. John's Wort can interact with some medicines, especially those taken to thin the blood. If taking prescribed medicines, consult your doctor or herbalist before taking St. John's Wort.

Dosage: flowering tops
Infusion   – 2g per cup: up to 3 cups a day
Capsule   – up to 2g a day
Tablet   – as recommended on label (generally up to 1000 mcg hypericin standardised extract a day)
Tincture (1:3) – up to 10 ml a day

Combinations:
With Black Cohosh for menopausal problems in general, especially when associated with nervous exhaustion and long-term stress
With Kava or Scullcap for anxiety, lowered mood and disturbed sleep
With Echinacea and Elderflower/berry for frequent or chronic viral infections

Scullcap ~ *Scutellaria laterifolia*

Key uses: Anxiety, nervous exhaustion, stress and stress-related symptoms such as headache, nervous tension and irritability, insomnia, pre-menstrual tension.

Uses during menopause: Scullcap has much to offer as a calming and soothing herb for nervous and stress-related problems in general. During the menopause, it is likely to find most use whenever anxiety and nervous exhaustion are a part of the picture – the nervousness or anxiety that can accompany hot-flushes, general irritability and unprovoked anger, and a proneness to crying can all be eased. With a dual ability to relax and tone the nervous system, Scullcap is a specific for nervous problems resulting from long-term stress – problems which can become prominent around the time of the menopause. Tension headaches, difficulty in concentrating, disturbed or restless sleep, general unhappiness and that sense of not being able to settle – all can benefit from Scullcap's soothing embrace. It combines well with Kava Kava, especially in anxiety, panic attacks and insomnia. A North American herb, the Cherokee took it to stimulate menstruation and ease breast pain, and it makes an effective remedy for pre-menstrual problems including breast tenderness and nervous irritability, as well as for spasmodic period pains.

Other uses: Scullcap's gently bitter taste indicates that the herb is a rounded tonic, stimulating digestion as well as nervous function, and thereby strengthening body and mind as a whole. Scullcap is mildly cooling and takes 'heat' out of stressful situations. As a nervine (nerve tonic) it is indicated for a wide range of nervous and nerve-related disorders including shock, overwork and chronic fatigue. Traditionally, Scullcap has been seen as a herb with a 'deeper' action on the nervous system than almost any other, being prescribed by medical herbalists for convulsions, epilepsy and 'hysteria', as well as serious mental illness. Scullcap is also useful in relieving muscular tension and spasms.

Research: There has been almost no research into this useful North American plant.

Dosage: Aerial parts (3-4 year old plants)
Infusion   – up to 6g a day
Capsule   – up to 3g a day
Tablet   – usually in combination with Valerian and Passiflora
Tincture (1:5) – up to 15ml per day

Combinations:
With Liquorice and St. John's Wort for nervous exhaustion and depression
With Black Cohosh for headaches, irritability, anxiety and nervousness
With Kava Kava for panic attacks and insomnia
With Agnus Castus for pre-menstrual breast tenderness and period pains

Wild Yam ~ *Dioscorea villosa*

Key uses: Hormonal tonic; for cramps and spasms; chronic inflammation including arthritis.

Uses during menopause: Surprisingly, given its popularity as a treatment for menopausal disorders, Wild Yam has no traditional use for the menopause in its native Mexico and USA. Its current use as an alternative to HRT and a remedy for menopausal symptoms stems largely from its claimed progesterogenic activity (see *Research* below). Wild Yam is not progesterogenic but contains steroidal saponins which have an oestrogenic effect, and it can make a valuable addition in treating menopausal problems. Many herbalists find that it combines well with Black Cohosh – perhaps to support hormonal balance as a long term alternative to HRT, but also for arthritic problems that develop during the menopause, typically affecting the finger joints.

Other traditional uses: Wild Yam is a good anti-spasmodic and may be taken to relieve stomach and abdominal cramps, as well as the pains of irritable bowel syndrome. It can also be taken to relieve ovarian pains and period cramps. Thought to have notable anti-inflammatory activity, it has longstanding use in the treatment of inflammatory arthritis including rheumatoid arthritis – combine here with Devil's Claw and Black Cohosh.

Research: Wild Yam has oestrogenic activity and does not contain progesterone. Products available over the counter which describe themselves as 'Wild Yam natural progesterone cream' are, to put it kindly, misleading. The progesterone in such creams is slightly more 'natural' than synthetic progesterone but has even less connection with Wild Yam than aspirin has with Willow bark – the plant material from which aspirin-type substances were first isolated in the 19th century. That being said, many women have found that 'natural' progesterone patches used for a few months at a time can provide significant relief of menopausal symptoms such as hot flushing and irritability. Such an approach to treatment is probably best utilised if herbal treatment has proved unsuccessful. There has been almost no research into Wild Yam, though its oestrogenic constituents – steroidal saponins – were used to create the first contraceptive pills in the 1950's.

Dosage: root

Infusion   – up to 8g a day
Capsule   – up to 4g a day
Tablet   – as recommended by manufacturer
Tincture (1:5) – up to 15ml per day.

Combinations:

With Black Cohosh to promote hormonal balance and for inflammatory arthritis

With Chinese Angelica and Fenugreek to support hormonal balance at the menopause and for vaginal dryness and lowered libido

With Liquorice and Sage for abdominal cramps and irritable bowel syndrome

With Motherwort and/or Agnus Castus for premenstrual symptoms and period pains

6 | When to see a medical herbalist

One reason that herbal medicine has become so popular is that plant medicines are safer and cause fewer side effects than conventional medicines. Through their ability to encourage normal, balanced function and to strengthen the body's self-repairing processes, herbal remedies are well suited to treating many health problems, particularly chronic 'disorders' – where the body and mind have lost the capacity to restore healthy balance and function.

In simple and relatively mild health problems, self-treatment with herbal medicine can be effective and safe. Taking Elderflower tea or Elderberry extract to treat a cold or flu can cut recovery time by 50%. Similarly, taking Black Cohosh for mild to moderate hot flushing or disordered temperature regulation can bring quick relief in symptoms.

Where menopausal symptoms are more severe, or have been going on for several months, or where you experience no improvement in symptoms on taking over the counter herbal remedies, it makes sense to consult a qualified medical herbalist. S/he will be able to give sound advice on diet and lifestyle changes that may help and will select herbal medicines appropriate for your condition and your constitution.

Medical herbalists also have knowledge of, and access to, a range of more potent medicinal plants, and while it is very likely that some of the herbs listed in this book will be appropriate, others may be prescribed that are not available over the counter. Consulting a medical herbalist will cost more in the short term but, by providing good quality herbs selected individually for each person, may well save money in the long term.

Consult a medical herbalist or your GP for advice on treating menopausal problems, where:

- you have self-treated with herbs for four or more weeks and no improvement has occurred

- you feel worse for taking a herbal medicine (discontinue treatment immediately if you feel worse – and contact a medical herbalist or your GP)
- you have allergies or are prone to allergic or unexpected reactions to foods or medicines
- you are already taking conventional medicines (usually it is fine to take herbal medicines at the same time as conventional medicines but it makes sense to seek advice in this situation)
- you have other significant health problems besides menopausal symptoms

7 | Further information

Further reading

Menopause: the Natural Way Molly Siple and Deborah Gordon, Wiley (2001)

The Menopause, HRT and You Caroline Hawkridge, Penguin (1999)

Sage Penelope Ody, Souvenir Press (2000)

Phytotherapy – Fifty Vital Herbs Andrew Chevallier, Amberwood (1998)

Encyclopedia of Medicinal Plants Andrew Chevallier, Dorling Kindersley (2001)

The Woman's Guide to Herbal Medicine Carol Rogers, Hamish Hamilton (1995)

Women Medicine: Vitex agnus castus Simon Mills, Amberwood (1992).

Contact Addresses

Amarant Trust
11-13 Charterhouse Buildings, London EC1M 7AN
Advice line on menopause counselling – 0891 660620

Continence Foundation
307 Hatton Square, 16 Baldwins Gardens, London EC1N 7RJ
Advice and information on continence including pelvic floor exercises
– 020 7404 6875

British Acupuncture Council
63 Jeddo Road, London W12 9HQ
Provides list of registered acupuncturists
– 020 8735 0400 – www.acupuncture.org.uk

Foundation for Integrated Medicine
International House, 59 Compton Road, London N1 2YT
Provides information on integrated medical services available in the NHS
– 020 7688 1881 – www.fimed.org

National Institute of Medical Herbalists
56 Longbrook St , Exeter EX4 6AH
Provides list of registered herbal practitioners
– 01392 426022 – www.nimh.org.uk

National Osteoporosis Society
PO Box 10, Radstock, Bath BA3 3YB
Helpline: 01761 472721

Register of Chinese Herbal Medicine
Office 5, Ferndale Business Centre, 1 Exeter Street, Norwich NR2 4QB
Provides list of registered Chinese herbal medicine practitioners
– www.rchm.co.uk

Royal London Homeopathic Hospital
Queen's Square, London WC1
Provides integrated medical treatment within the NHS - referral by a GP required

Society of Homeopaths
2 Artizan Road, Northampton NN1 4HU
Provides list of registered homeopaths
– www.homeopathy-soh.org

Women's Health – Resource and information centre
52 Featherstone Street, London EC1Y 8RT
Health Enquiry Line: 020 7251 6580

Women's Nutritional Advisory Service Ltd
PO Box 268, Lewes, E. Sussex BN7 2QN
01273 487366 / Fax 01273 487576
E-mail: wnas@org.uk

Other Websites
Medline Plus – http://www.nlm.nih.gov/medlineplus

8 | Index of herbs

OTHER BOOKS FROM AMBERWOOD PUBLISHING ARE:

Aromatherapy Lexicon – The Essential Reference by Geoff Lyth and Sue Charles is a colourful, fun way to learn about Aromatherapy. £4.99.

Aromatherapy – The Baby Book by Marion Del Gaudio Mak. An easy to follow guide to massage for the infant or child. £3.99

Aromatherapy – Simply For You by Marion Del Gaudio Mak. A clear, simple and comprehensive guide to Aromatherapy for beginners. £2.99.

Aromatherapy – A Guide for Home Use by Christine Westwood. All you need to know about essential oils and using them. £1.99.

Aromatherapy – for Stress Management by Christine Westwood. Covering the use of essential oils for everyday stress-related problems. £3.50.

Aromatherapy – For Healthy Legs and Feet by Christine Westwood. A guide to the use of essential oils for the treatment of legs and feet. £2.99.

Aromatherapy – The Pregnancy Book by Jennie Supper RM RN MGCP. Jennie Supper, a State Registered Nurse and Midwife explains the use of Aromatherapy during pregnancy and the common conditions which may be treated safely. £5.99

Aromatherapy – A Nurses Guide by Ann Percival SRN. The ultimate, safe, lay guide to the natural benefits of Aromatherapy. Including recipes and massage techniques for many medical conditions and a quick reference chart. £2.99.

Aromatherapy – A Nurses Guide for Women by Ann Percival SRN. Concentrates on women's health for all ages. Including sections on PMT, menopause, infertility, cellulite. £2.99.

Aromatherapy – Essential Oils in Colour by Rosemary Caddy Bsc Hons, ARCS MISP is a unique book depicting the chemistry of essential oils. £9.99.

Aroma Science – The Chemistry & Bioactivity of Essential Oils by Dr Maria Lis-Balchin. With a comprehensive list of the Oils and scientific analysis. Includes sections on the sense of smell and the history of Aromatherapy. £5.99.

Woman Medicine – Vitex Agnus Castus by Simon Mills MA, FNIMH. The story of the herb that has been used for centuries in the treatment of women's problems. £2.99.

Plant Medicine – A Guide for Home Use (New Edition) by Charlotte Mitchell MNIMH. A guide to home use giving an insight into the wonderful healing qualities of plants. £2.99.

Ancient Medicine – Ginkgo Biloba (New Edition) by Dr Desmond Corrigan BSc(Pharms), MA, Phd, FLS, FPSI. Improved memory, circulation and concentration are associated with Ginkgo and explained in this book. £2.99.

Indian Medicine – The Immune System by Dr Desmond Corrigan BSc(Pharms), MA, Phd, FLS, FPSI. An intriguing account of the history of the plant called Echinacea and its power to influence the immune system. £2.99.

Herbal Medicine for Sleep & Relaxation by Dr Desmond Corrigan BSc(Pharms), MA, PhD, FLS, FPSI. A guide to the natural sedatives as an alternative to orthodox drug therapies, drawing on the latest medical research, presented in an easy reference format. £2.99.

Herbal First Aid by Andrew Chevallier BA, MNIMH. A beautifully clear reference book of natural remedies and general first aid in the home. £3.50.

Natural Taste – Herbal Teas, A Guide for Home Use by Andrew Chevallier BA, MNIMH. Contains a comprehensive compendium of Herbal Teas gives information on how to make it, its benefits, history and folklore. £3.50.

Garlic– How Garlic Protects Your Heart by Prof E. Ernst MD, PhD. Used as a medicine for over 4500 years, this book examines the latest scientific evidence supporting Garlic's effect in reducing cardiovascular disease, the Western World's number one killer. £3.99.

Phytotherapy – Fifty Vital Herbs by Andrew Chevallier, the most popular medicinal herbs with uses and advice written by an expert. £6.99

Insomnia – Doctor I Can't Sleep by Dr Adrian Williams FRCP. Written by one of the world's leading sleep experts, Dr Williams explains the phenomenon of sleep and sleeping disorders and gives advice on treatment. With 25% of the adult population reporting difficulties sleeping – this book will be essential reading for many. £2.99.

Eyecare Eyewear – For Better Vision by Mark Rossi Bsc, MBCO. A complete guide to eyecare and eyewear including an assessment of the types of spectacles and contact lenses available and the latest corrective surgical procedures. £3.99.

Arthritis and Rheumatism by Dr John Cosh FRCP, MD. Covers all forms of Arthritis, its effects and the treatments available. £4.95.

All You Ever Wanted To Know About Vitamins by Dr Leonard Mervyn. The ultimate book on nutrition. £6.99.